HOW FITNESS HELPS WITH MENTAL HEALTH

FITNESS TACTICS FOR HANDLING MENTAL HEALTH ISSUES

AHMED .R

Contents

CHAPTER ONE

Introduction

In a time when anxiety and stress are common, many people now place a high priority on maintaining their mental health. Although conventional methods such as counseling and medication are still important, getting fit is a popular way to support mental health.

Numerous forms of physical activity have been praised for their ability to both shape bodies and develop minds. In order to better understand the mutually beneficial relationship between fitness and mental health, this introduction will look at the many ways that regular exercise can improve emotional and psychological well-being.

The Relationship Between the Mind and Body

Ancient philosophies and healing traditions have long stressed the interdependence of physical and mental health, so the idea of a mind-body link is not new. This idea is still supported by contemporary research, which clarifies the complex processes by which physical exercise affects mental health and emotional stability.

Impact on Neurobiology

A series of neurobiological alterations brought about by exercise support mental health. The body's natural mood enhancers, endorphins, are released when physical activity occurs, and this influence extends to the regulation of neurotransmitters such as dopamine and serotonin.

Reduction of Stress and Resilience

The capacity to control and reduce stress is essential for maintaining mental health in a world full of pressures. Frequent exercise is a powerful way to combat stress because it provides a healthy way to release stored up energy and builds resilience in the face of hardship.

Improved Mental Abilities

Fitness has been demonstrated to improve cognitive function and guard against cognitive decline in addition to its effects on mood. Exercise strengthens mental acuity by enhancing neuroplasticity, or the brain's capacity to adapt and remodel itself. It also improves cognitive flexibility, memory retention, and executive function.

Social Cohesion and Assistance

For many people, the gym or yoga studio is a hub for social contact and community involvement rather than merely a place to work out physically. Shared exercise relationships can create a sense of community and support, acting as a preventative measure against the prevalent ills of modern life—loneliness and isolation.

Independence and Self-Sufficiency

Starting a fitness journey fosters self-efficacy and empowerment, or the conviction that one can bring about positive change. Setting and completing fitness objectives boosts self-esteem and confidence in people, creating a resilient mindset that goes beyond the gym.

It is impossible to overestimate the importance of fitness and mental health in the pursuit of complete well-being. People who make the most of their physical activity can improve their cognitive abilities, develop emotional fortitude, and create relationships that uplift their spirits.

Let's acknowledge the transforming power of exercise as a foundational element of mental wellness as we begin our exploration.

the significance of mental wellness

Mental well-being is crucial for a number of reasons:

General Well-Being: One essential element of general well-being is mental health. It includes social, psychological, and emotional health. Neglecting one's mental health can result in a number of problems, such as stress, anxiety, depression, and other mental diseases.

Quality of Life: An individual's quality of life is greatly enhanced by having good mental health. It enables people to deal with life's challenges, keep happy relationships, work efficiently, and partake in enjoyable and satisfying activities.

Physical Health: There is a close relationship between mental and physical health. Physical and mental health can be adversely impacted by one another. Chronic stress, for instance, can impair immunity and raise the risk of a number of physical health conditions, including obesity, digestive disorders, and cardiovascular illnesses.

Productivity: In both personal and professional life, mental health is a critical factor in performance and productivity. People who are in good mental health are more adept at focusing, making decisions, problem-solving, and accomplishing their objectives.

Relationships: Strong mental health is the cornerstone of a healthy relationship. People who are in good mental health are better able to express empathy, communicate clearly, settle disputes, and build strong relationships with others.

Resilience: The capacity to overcome adversity, adjust to change, and recover from setbacks is largely dependent on one's mental health. People who possess resilience are better able to manage life's obstacles and come out stronger from trying circumstances.

Decreased stigma: Increasing mental well-being contributes to a less stigmatized mental health environment. A more accepting and encouraging environment is produced for all when society recognizes the value of mental health and provides assistance to those who are struggling with mental health concerns.

Economic Impact: There are major financial ramifications for mental health. Reduced productivity, absenteeism, higher healthcare expenditures, and a burden on social services are all possible outcomes of mental health issues. Long-term financial gains and cost reductions can result from spending money on mental health promotion and treatment.

All things considered, the well-being of people, groups, and civilizations depends on giving mental health first priority. It necessitates an all-encompassing strategy that takes into account early intervention, prevention, access to high-quality mental health treatment, and the development of supportive environments that promote mental health.

Comprehending Mental Health

Recognizing the complexity of the human mind and how it influences feelings, ideas, actions, and general well-being is essential to understanding mental health. Here are a few crucial elements to take into account when attempting to comprehend mental health:

Biopsychosocial Model: Social, psychological, and biological aspects all have an impact on mental health. A few examples of biological influences are physical health, mental chemistry, and heredity. Emotions, personality traits, and cognitive processes are examples of psychological factors. Relationships, financial status, culture, and pressures in the environment are all considered social factors. Comprehending mental health necessitates taking into account the interaction of these diverse elements.

Normal Variation: There is a continuum of mental health, from perfect wellbeing to mental disease. It is important to understand that worry, sadness, and anxiety are natural emotions and do not always signify a mental health issue. On the other hand, severe or chronic symptoms that make it difficult to go about daily tasks could call for medical treatment.

Resilience: The capacity to overcome hardship and preserve mental health in the face of difficulties is known as resilience. Although some people might be more resilient by nature, resilience can also be developed via self-care routines, coping mechanisms, and supportive connections.

Stigma: The stigma associated with mental illness can exacerbate preconceived notions, prejudice, and obstacles to getting treatment. In order to understand mental health, one must fight stigma and advance inclusivity, empathy, and compassion for those who suffer from mental illnesses.

Risk and Protective Factors: A number of variables, including trauma, a family history of mental illness, long-term stress, substance misuse, and social isolation, raise the possibility of developing mental health issues. On the other hand, protective variables can increase resilience and function as a buffer against mental health issues. These include strong social support, constructive coping mechanisms, availability to mental health care, and a supportive environment.

Prevention and Early Intervention: Proactive approaches can help to improve mental health in the same way that they can improve physical health via habits like regular exercise and a balanced diet. It is possible to delay the onset of mental illness and lessen its effects by promoting mental health literacy, providing coping skills education, creating supportive communities, and addressing sociocultural factors that influence mental health.

Holistic Approach to Treatment: Biological, psychological, and social aspects must all be taken into consideration while treating mental health conditions. This could entail individualized self-care routines, social support networks, medication, therapy, and lifestyle modifications.

Cultural Considerations: Mental health experiences and manifestations differ between cultures, and it is essential to comprehend these differences in order to provide care that is sensitive to cultural differences. diverse cultures have diverse perspectives on, experiences with, and approaches to mental health according to cultural beliefs, norms, values, and resource accessibility.

Through these lenses, people and communities may better support mental health, lessen stigma, and encourage everyone's resilience and recovery by developing a deeper understanding of mental health.

Fitness's Significance for Mental Health

Fitness through a variety of physiological, psychological, and social pathways contributes significantly to the promotion of mental health and well-being. The following are some ways that physical fitness supports mental health:

Endorphin Release: Engaging in physical activity triggers the brain's natural painkiller and mood enhancer, endorphins, to be released. Exercise-induced endorphin releases can lower stress and anxiety levels and produce euphoric feelings.

Stress Reduction: Engaging in regular physical activity aids in lowering the body's cortisol levels, which are a sign of stress. Exercise can be a healthy way to release tension, stress, and pent-up energy, which can help you feel calmer and more at ease.

Exercise has been demonstrated to increase the quantity and quality of sleep, which is crucial for mental health.

CHAPTER TWO

While sleep interruptions are associated with an increased risk of mood disorders like sadness and anxiety, adequate sleep supports cognitive function, emotional regulation, and general well-being.

Brain Health: Exercise increases neuroplasticity, or the brain's capacity to change and rearrange itself. Frequent exercise has been linked to increased cognitive function, which includes better decision-making, memory, and focus. Additionally, it aids in defending against neurodegenerative illnesses including Alzheimer's and age-related cognitive decline.

Increased Self-esteem: Participating in physical activity and reaching fitness objectives can increase one's sense of confidence and self-worth. Frequent exercise promotes a sense of success, competence and mastery, and a favorable body image—all of which are beneficial to mental health and a positive self-perception.

Social Interaction: Whether it's through team sports, group exercise programs, or outdoor leisure activities, social interaction is a big part of many fitness activities. Engaging in social interactions while exercising offers chances for bonding, encouragement, and teamwork—all of which are crucial for psychological well-being and a feeling of inclusion.

Exercise is a healthy diversion from worry, negative thoughts, and rumination. It also helps with coping. By changing attention and fostering mindfulness, physical activity offers a momentary reprieve from pressures and aids in the management of challenging emotions.

Mood Regulation: Regular exercise helps reduce the symptoms of anxiety and sadness by having a mood-regulating effect. Serotonin and dopamine, two neurotransmitters important for motivation, pleasure, and mood control, can be elevated by it.

Benefits for Long-Term Mental Health: Developing a regular fitness regimen can have a positive impact on mental health over the long run by lowering the risk of mental diseases including depression and anxiety disorders. Being physically healthy helps people be more resilient overall, which makes it easier for them to handle life's obstacles and preserve their mental health.

In general, sustaining excellent mental health and fostering general well-being depend heavily on include regular physical activity into one's lifestyle. Fittingness can have a significant positive impact on mental health, whether it is achieved through organized exercise regimens, leisure pursuits, or just staying active all day.

Fitness Activities Types for Mental Wellness

Fitness activities come in a variety of forms that can improve mental health by elevating general quality of life, lowering stress, elevating physical well-being, and increasing mood. Here are a few instances:

Cardiovascular Work:

Running/Jogging: Besides increasing cardiovascular fitness and producing endorphins, running or jogging outside can give one a sense of independence and a connection to the natural world.

Cycling: Cycling is a low-impact aerobic activity that may be done alone or in groups. It can be done on a stationary bike or outside. Cycling also promotes cardiovascular health.

Swimming: A great way to relieve tension and revitalize the mind, swimming is a full-body exercise that is easy on the joints and encourages relaxation.

Strengthening Exercise:

Weightlifting: Exercises that increase muscular strength and endurance, posture, and confidence can be performed with free weights, resistance bands, or weight machines.

Bodyweight Exercises: Bodyweight exercises are great for keeping up physical and mental health because they are portable and require little equipment, such push-ups, squats, and lunges.

Mind-Body Practices:

Yoga: Yoga promotes relaxation, flexibility, and stress reduction by combining physical postures, breathing exercises, and mindfulness activities. It has been demonstrated to raise general mental health, lessen anxiety, and increase mood.

Pilates: Through deliberate movements and breath work, Pilates focuses on body awareness, flexibility, and core strength. It can enhance mental focus, balance, and posture.

Tai Chi: With its calm, flowing movements and in-depth breathing, Tai Chi is a gentle martial art. It is advantageous for stress management and mental health since it fosters balance, relaxation, and mental clarity.

Outdoor Pursuits:

Hiking: Hiking in the outdoors offers the therapeutic advantages of being outside, such as lowered stress levels, elevated moods, and increased cognitive performance, in addition to physical activity.

Rock Climbing: This physical and mental challenge calls for tenacity, focus, and problem-solving abilities. It can increase self-assurance, resiliency, and a feeling of achievement.

Group Exercise Programs:

Dance-Based Fitness Classes: Classes that combine aerobic exercise with rhythmic movement and music, like Zumba or hip-hop dance, encourage happiness, self-expression, and social interaction.

Group Exercise: Instructor-led structured workouts in a motivating group setting are offered in group fitness courses like aerobics, spinning, or circuit training. These classes promote motivation, accountability, and camaraderie.

Combat Sports and Martial Arts:

Martial arts disciplines, such as Karate, Judo, or Tae Kwon Do, emphasize self-defense techniques, discipline, and physical conditioning. They also foster mental toughness, emotional control, and self-confidence.

Boxing or Kickboxing: These fitness regimens mix strength training, cardio, and stress release through punching and kicking techniques, enhancing mood and empowering people.

Sports for Recreation:

Tennis, Basketball, Soccer: By friendly competition and teamwork, team sports and leisure leagues offer chances for physical activity, social engagement, and stress release.

Whatever the exact fitness activity selected, adding regular exercise to one's regimen can significantly improve mental health and enhance general wellbeing and quality of life.

Fitting Exercise Into Everyday Living

Maintaining general health and well-being requires integrating fitness into daily living. The following are some doable methods for working exercise into your everyday schedule:

Establish Achievable Fitness Goals That Fit Your Interests, Preferences, and Current Fitness Level: First, establish realistic fitness goals. Whether your goal is to complete a fitness challenge, work out for 30 minutes three times a week, or walk 10,000 steps a day, setting and meeting specific goals will help you stay motivated and accountable.

Set Aside Time for Exercise: Allocate specific time on your daily or weekly calendar for physical activity, just as you would any other important appointment. Whether it's in the morning, during lunch breaks, or in the evening, figure out when it's most convenient for you to exercise, and try your best to keep to your workout routine.

Discover Exercises You Love: Try out a variety of physical pursuits and decide which ones you actually enjoy and eagerly anticipate engaging in. It is simpler to stick to a fitness plan when you include enjoyable activities such as walking, cycling, dancing, swimming, yoga, or gardening.

Make It Easy: Seek methods to incorporate exercise into your everyday routine that are both easier and more convenient. This may be working out at home using fitness apps or online workout videos, signing up for a local gym or studio, or employing active commuting options like cycling or walking in place of driving.

Integrate Exercise with Daily Routines: Make the most of your time by combining physical activity with your regular tasks and routines. For instance, walk or bike instead of driving to local locations, use the stairs instead of the elevator, or perform bodyweight exercises while watching TV or while waiting for food to prepare.

Divide It Up: If scheduling a single, long workout session is difficult, divide up your activity into smaller, more manageable sessions spread out throughout the day. Short bursts of exercise, such brisk bodyweight circuits or ten-minute walks, can build up and improve your general fitness.

Include Others: To make exercise more fun and social, go with friends, family, or coworkers.

Taking part in team sports, forming a walking club, or enrolling in a group fitness class can offer you the inspiration, accountability, and support you need to maintain your fitness objectives.

create Reminders and Track success: You may create reminders, track your activity levels, and track your success over time by using technological tools like wearables, smartphone apps, and fitness trackers. Observing your successes and turning points could support you in reaffirming your resolve to keep forward.

Be Adaptable and Flexible: When it comes to your exercise regimen, be Adaptable and Flexible, especially when unforeseen circumstances or time restraints occur.

Recognize that days may come when your workout doesn't go as planned, and be prepared to modify your routine or activity level guilt-free.

Prioritize Self-Care: To support your fitness efforts and preserve balance in your life, remember that physical activity is only one component of overall well-being. Give self-care habits like getting enough sleep, eating a good diet, managing stress, and practicing relaxation techniques top priority.

You can make physical activity a fun and sustainable part of your routine by implementing these ideas into your daily life. This will improve your emotional and physical well-being as well as your overall fitness and health.

CHAPTER THREE

Overcoming Obstacles to Mental Health Fitness

Identifying typical challenges that may prevent people from participating in physical exercise and putting methods in place to overcome them are key to overcoming barriers to fitness for mental health. Here are some typical obstacles and solutions for them:

Absence of drive:

Make sure your exercise objectives are attainable, inspiring, and have personal significance.

To make working out more pleasurable and inspiring, find things you look forward to doing.

Get yourself a support system of friends, family, or fellow exercise enthusiasts who will inspire and motivate you.

Time Restrictions:

Divide up your daily exercise routine into shorter, more doable sessions, such bodyweight workouts or 10-minute walks.

Make physical activity a priority by blocking out time on your daily or weekly calendar for exercise.

Seek out opportunities to work out throughout your regular activities, such as doing housework, watching TV, or taking a lunch break.

Fatigue or a lack of energy:

As your energy levels rise, start with low-intensity exercises like walking or light stretching and progressively increase the intensity.

To make sure you're well-rested and have the energy to engage in physical exercise, prioritize getting enough sleep and maintain proper sleep hygiene.

Select pursuits that bring you a sense of renewal and energy, such vigorous yoga classes or strolls in the great outdoors.

Budgetary Restrictions:

Look into free or inexpensive ways to get fit, like going for a run or walk outside, using fitness apps or online tutorials, or taking part in group exercise sessions.

Check for special offers, promotions, or government-funded initiatives from nearby fitness establishments, gyms, or leisure centers.

Invest in reasonably priced workout tools or accessories, such jump ropes, yoga mats, or resistance bands, so you can work out at home.

Self-consciousness or issues with one's body image:

Select fitness pursuits or settings that make you feel welcome and at ease, such as personal training sessions at home or inclusive exercise programs.

Instead of concentrating just on looks or weight loss, consider the benefits of physical activity, such as enhanced health, mood, and energy levels.

Regardless of perceived shortcomings or limitations, acknowledge your efforts and progress to combat negative self-talk and cultivate self-compassion.

Limitations on the body or health issues:

Before beginning any new fitness program, speak with a healthcare provider, particularly if you have any underlying medical issues or physical restrictions.

Collaborate with a licensed fitness specialist, such as a physical therapist or personal trainer, who can customize workouts to meet your unique requirements, capabilities, and objectives.

Select low-impact or adapted workouts like chair yoga, water aerobics, or swimming that can suit physical restrictions and yet be beneficial to your health.

Climate or Environmental Elements:

When weather conditions prevent you from working outside, have a backup plan for working out indoors. This can include employing fitness classes, at-home training equipment, or indoor workout videos.

Make an investment in weather-appropriate gear and apparel, such as moisture-wicking clothes, waterproof shoes, or accessories for colder climates, so you can work out outside in comfort under a variety of circumstances.

Symptoms of Mental Health:

Acknowledge that engaging in physical activity can be an effective strategy for coping with mental health symptoms like stress, anxiety, or depression.

When you're feeling overwhelmed or tired, start with moderate, low-intensity exercises and work your way up to more intense ones when you feel up to it.

To improve relaxation and mental clarity before, during, or after exercise, practice mindfulness techniques like deep breathing or body scans.

You may establish a supportive environment that encourages regular physical activity, boosts mood, lowers stress levels, and improves general well-being by recognizing and removing barriers to fitness for mental health. As you travel the path of fitness, never forget to appreciate your accomplishments and to be kind and patient with yourself.

Summary

In conclusion, there is no denying the link between mental health and physical fitness, and engaging in regular physical activity has several advantages. In addition to improving physical health, fitness is essential for fostering resilience and mental wellness. People who exercise regularly report feeling happier, less stressed, having more self-esteem, and living a higher quality of life overall.

Fitness exercises like aerobics, strength training, and mind-body therapies like yoga and tai chi can have a significant impact on mental health by promoting neuroplasticity, lowering stress hormones, and releasing endorphins. In addition to offering chances for social connection, self-expression, relaxation, and personal development, these activities also promote a sense of fulfillment and purpose.

Fitness also provides a comprehensive approach to mental health treatment by addressing the social, psychological, and biological aspects of wellbeing. People can overcome obstacles including a lack of desire, time restraints, self-consciousness, and physical restrictions by integrating fitness into their daily lives. This allows them to develop long-lasting habits that promote resilience and mental health.

Essentially, exercise is a potent tool for improving mental health because it gives people the confidence to take charge of their health and develop a healthy relationship with their bodies and minds. People can harness physical activity's transforming ability to thrive emotionally, psychologically, and physically by realizing the tremendous impact it has on mental health and making it a priority in their self-care routines.

THE END